INTRODUCTION 2

WHY CAN SUGAR BE DANGEROUS? 7

EFFECTS ON HEART 9

HOW MUCH SUGAR CAN I EAT? 13

WHY IS SUGAR ADDICTIVE? 17

SIX TYPES OF SUGAR 20

HOW TO GET AWAY FROM SUGAR 24

AVOID ARTIFICIAL SUGAR 26

FOCUS ON WHOLE FOODS 27

SPICES TO EAT 29

ALTERNATIVES TO SUGAR 31

RECIPES WITHOUT SUGAR 35

COCONUT BISCUITS (SMALL) 35

COCONUT LEMONS BISCUITS 37

CHOCOLATE CHERRIE CAKE 40

PEANUT BUTTER PROTEIN PANCAKES............................44

SUGAR-FREE MUFFINS 50

SNACK WITH BERRIES AND CHIA SEEDS 57

CONCLUSION..59

Sugar free nutrition

Life without sugar

Denise Bergmann

Hello and welcome! This guide will tell you why sugar is harmful, why it is so addictive, how to detect and avoid sugar addiction, and how you can try to live without sugar. It's not that hard as you think. I'll also explain what are the alternatives to sugars. To succeed in a sugar-free diet, you only need consistency and stamina nothing more! I am glad that you read this book and hope to be able to help you with getting your sugar addiction behind.

Harmful Sugars

There are many different types of sugar, almost flooding the market. The question is, of course, which type of sugar should I take? Are there really better sugars than others? Whether honey, coconut sugar, or the classic deadly white sugar. All of these sweeteners are sugar supply mechanisms with little difference. Some are fructose, others are sucrose and affect the body in different ways.

Fructose is a type of sugar known as monosaccharide. Sucrose, on the other hand, is a disaccharide. It is broken down into glucose and fructose before it enters the bloodstream and raises blood sugar levels. Increases blood sugar levels damage blood vessels and lead among others to tooth decay and gum disease.

Fructose does not enter the bloodstream like glucose. It must go first to the liver, where it is used, in order not to raise the blood sugar level. When you consume excess calories and fructose, fructose is converted to triglycerides.

In this case it is even more harmful than glucose. Fructose is beneficial in restoring glycogen, which is an important saturation signal for the brain. In addition, fructose causes less caries and gum disease.

On the whole it can be said that no sugar is necessarily better than the other. Too much sugar in the form of glucose, sucrose, or fructose can lead to all of the above-mentioned problems. The effect on your health depends on how much you consume from the sugar.

Mainly the following types of sugar are used:

GRANULATED WHITE SUGAR

Type: sucrose

Advantages: White sugar is made from sugar cane or sugar beet. It has the mildest taste, melts and mixes easily with hot or cold drinks and is ideal for baking.

Disadvantages: This type of sugar undergoes the strongest chemical processing.

ASPARTAME

Type: artificial substitute

Advantages: Sugar free and no calories

Disadvantages: This sweetener consists of chemical compounds. It is not nutritious. Actually, aspartame is on a list of potential carcinogens in many countries, including Germany. In animal studies, high doses of this substance are associated with leukaemia.

BROWN SUGAR

Type: sucrose

Advantages: After processing is part of the molasses, which is left over from the refining process, put into the sugar, which provides a small amount of micro-nutrients.

Disadvantages: Not many nutrients remain.

Why can sugar be dangerous?

Of course, sugar is present in all foods that contain carbohydrates, such as fruits, vegetables, grains and dairy products. The consumption of whole foods with natural sugar is fine. Plant foods also have high levels of fiber, essential minerals and antioxidants. Dairy products contain protein and calcium. As your body slowly digests these foods, the sugar provides a steady supply of energy to your cells. High intake of fruits, vegetables and whole grains has been proven to reduce the risk of chronic diseases such as diabetes, heart disease and some cancer.

Problems caused by too much sugar intake

However, problems occur when you ingest too much sugar, which is sugar that food manufacturers add to products to improve taste.

The worst sources of sugar are soft drinks, fruit drinks, flavored yoghurts, cereals, biscuits, cakes, sweets and most processed foods.

The result: we consume too much sugar. Adult men consume an average of 20 teaspoons of sugar a day, equivalent to 330 calories.

The influence of excess sugar on obesity and diabetes is well documented. However, one area that will surprise many men is how their cravings for sugar can have a serious impact on their heart health.

A study published in Austria in 2013 showed (link given below) people dying because of a high-sugar intake and a higher risk of dying from heart disease. Over the 10-year study, people who received 19% to 29% of their calories from added sugar had a 38% higher risk of dying from cardiovascular disease than those who received 9% of their calories as extra sugar.

<u>Basically, higher the addition of sugar have higher the risk of heart disease.</u>

How sugar actually affect heart health, is not yet entirely clear, but appears to have several indirect connections. For example, large amounts of sugar overload the liver. Your liver uses sugar in the same way as alcohol and converts dietary carbohydrates into fat. Over time, this can lead to increase accumulation of fat, which can lead to fatty liver disease, which contributes to diabetes and increases the risk of heart disease.

Too much sugar can increase blood pressure and increase chronic inflammation, both pathological pathways to heart disease. Excessive sugar intake, especially in sugary drinks, also contributes to weight gain, causing your body to turn off its appetite suppressant system, as liquid calories are not as satisfying as solid food calories. For this reason, it is easier for people to add more calories to their normal diet when consuming sugary drinks.

The effects of extra sugar intake is high blood pressure, inflammation, weight gain, diabetes and fatty liver - are all associated with an increased risk of heart attack and stroke. In addition, sugar causes overweight, which today has become a real epidemic in many countries. It is not the only "culprit", but plays a major role. What are the side effect? For example, if you consume fructose, it triggers a rather atypical insulin response. Fructose is deposited directly in the liver. It becomes fat instead of glycogen. Basically, it tells the body, "Save fat and stay hungry".

The food industry aggravates a certain problem, namely to fight against the calorie intake. We assume that you need to use less calories if you want to lose weight. That's not true, because not all calories are the same.

What is the purpose of this approach? People forgo 500 calories of a healthy food, such as pecans, to eat a 500-calorie chocolate bar.

It is important to note that sugar causes chronic degenerative diseases.

The consumption of sugar is strongly related to diabetes, high blood pressure, heart disease, obesity and even cancer and Alzheimer's. It nourishes and promotes almost every disease process, including Candida. Cancer cells like sugar, as do viruses, fungi, mold, bacteria, parasites, and yeasts. These baddies thrive on sugar and acid, which is also formed by sugar.

If 20 teaspoons of sugar per day is too much, what is the right amount?

It's hard to say because sugar is not a necessary nutrient in your diet. Experts suggest that we should not consume more than 140 calories (about 8 teaspoons or 32 grams) of sugar per day. This is close to the amount in a can of soda.

Reading food labels is one of the best ways to control the intake of sugar.

Look for the following extra sugar names and try to avoid or reduce the amount and they are found in:

- Honey
- Molasses
- Brown sugar
- Corn syrup

- Corn sweetener

- Concentrated fruit juices

- Corn syrup with high fructose content

- Malt sugar

- Syrup sugar molecules that end in "ose" (dextrose, fructose, glucose, lactose, maltose, sucrose).

The total content of sugar, including additional sugars, is often given in grams.

Write down the number of grams of sugar per serving as well as the total number of servings. It could only be 3 grams of sugar per serving, but if the normal amount is ten or twelve servings, that's over 30 grams of sugar of your daily limit.

Also, keep an eye on the sugar you add to your food or drink. About half of the added sugar comes from beverages, including coffee and tea. A 2017 study found that about two thirds of coffee drinkers and one third of tea drinkers add sugar or sugary substances to their drinks.

The researchers also found that more than 70% of the calories in their drinks came from added sugar.

But experts warn against overeating in their attempts to reduce sugar, as this can lead to false reactions. You may be looking for other foods to satisfy your hunger for something sweet, such as refined starches like white bread and white rice that can raise your glucose levels, and foods that are high in saturated fat and sodium this also one of the causes for heart problems.

Do you know that sugar is ten times more addictive than cocaine? It affects the same regions of the brain as cocaine and heroin. Specific people are hired by candy manufacturers to ensure that the products make consumers addicted. These people are paid to prepare "addictive, delicious, processed ready meals" with the aim of gaining the largest market share. Actually, sugar is nothing more than poison, which the body can process in small quantities.

Over time, our tolerance for sugar increases and we need more and more of it to achieve the same effects.

Animal studies have shown that animals who have suffered an electric shock, still consumed sugar during the impact. What do you think -

would a person continue to snort cocaine under such pressure?

Many scientists suggest that sugar plays a vital role in our survival. That is why we long for him (at least most of us). Our sense of taste has evolved to covet the vital molecules like salt, fat and sugar.

When we eat, the simple sugar glucose is absorbed by the intestine into the bloodstream and distributed to all cells of the body. Glucose is particularly important for the brain as it is an important source of billions of neuronal neurons.

Neurons need a constant supply from the bloodstream because they cannot store glucose themselves. As diabetics know, someone with low blood sugar can quickly go into a coma.

It's strange, but scientists have found that even the taste of sugar can give our brain a boost. Tests have shown that participants who saturate sugar sweetened water around their mouth respond better to mental tasks than if they were taking artificially sweetened water.

Six types of sugar

• **Glucose**: Simple sugar that can be transported in the blood.

• **Fructose**: Simple sugar that occurs naturally in fruits.

• **Sucrose**: Commonly known as table sugar, naturally occurs in sugar cane

• **Lactose**: Milk sugar, which contains less than 5% cow's milk

• **Maltose**: Two connected glucose molecules

• **High fructose** (corn syrup): Corn syrup, in which half of the glucose was converted to fructose. Chemically very similar to sucrose.

Our relationship with sugar will starts at birth because in that point itself we will have sweet tooth.

A recent study found that newborns have a pronounced preference for sweet flavours over other flavours. Even children enjoy sugary foods even more than adults.

Many scientists believe that a child's preference for sweet things is an evolutionary 'hangover', as adolescents who in former times favoured high-calorie foods would have better chances of survival if food sources were unreliable.

The problem now is that refined sugar is too readily available. This may be part of the reason why childhood obesity rates (obesity) have increased.

Doctors now recommend that parents avoid giving babies sweet food or drink to prevent them from getting a taste for them early in life.

Eating too much sugar can lead to unhealthy eating habits. Sugar can improve one's mood as it encourages the body to release the "endorphin hormone" serotonin into the bloodstream.

The immediate "boost," we get from sugar, is one of the reasons why we access candy when we are sad or unhappy. However, the pleasant feeling triggers an increase in insulin, as the body strives to bring the blood sugar level back to normal. As a result, we have a "sugar crash". That is why many crave more sugar, which can lead to a cycle of binge eating.

We just do not know when to stop

In addition, the body can't tell when we have to stop the sugars. Researchers have found that

foods and beverages sweetened with simple
fructose do not produce the same satiety as other
foods with similar calories. One study found that
while glucose suppresses the parts of the brain
that force us to eat; Fructose is not. The panellists
also reported that they felt happier after
consuming glucose compared to fructose. When
these two aspects are present, the risk increases
accordingly.

Here are 7 tips to get away from the sugar.

Take your time

One of the most important things to consider when changing your diet is to do it gradually. It should be a slow process from a diet full of sugar to sugar free diet.

It can help to eliminate the most obvious sources of sugar. Baked foods such as cakes, muffins and brownies can be easily avoided.

The elimination of sweets and sugary drinks is an excellent start.

You can also try to reduce the amount of sugar and cream you put into your coffee or tea, gradually eliminating it altogether. Working up to a sugar-free diet can help to re-train the palate, so no longer you miss sugar.

Avoid simple carbohydrates

Many sugar-free diets also recommends the people to avoid simple carbohydrates. The simple carbohydrates are white flour, white noodles and white rice.

The carbohydrates in these foods can be broken down in the body quickly to sugar, which rises the blood sugar level in the body. A person can substitute simple carbohydrates with whole grain options.

Avoid artificial sugar

Artificial sugar is a subject of controversy in the diet industry. They are much sweeter than sugar but contain little or no calories. Acceptance of artificial sugar can cause the body to believe that he actually consumed sugar. This can make a person's sugar hunger worse, which makes it harder for them to stick to a sugar-free diet.

Avoid/stop Sugar Drinks

Sugar is easily avoided in processed foods, but sweetened beverages such as soda, coffees, sweetened teas, and fruit juices are among the major sources of added sugars in the diet.

Replace these drinks with unsweetened herbal tea, coffee without sugar, mineral water or spring water. This can help you to reduce your sugar intake and stay hydrated.

Focus on whole foods

A person who does not consume sugar can also eat 100 percent whole foods. Processed foods contain more refined ingredients or added sugars. A diet with a focus on whole foods is as follows:

- Vegetables
- Fruits
- Lean meat, poultry or tofu
- Fish
- Whole, unprocessed grains and legumes
- Nuts and seeds

In addition, you can add dairy products to your meal plan.

Plan your meals

It is difficult to stick to a diet without a plan. When cravings occur, you are likely to grab unhealthy snacks as if you have a well-planned meal and know when to eat again to endure the cravings.

Many people spend a day preparing their purchases and meals for the entire week. When prepared, fewer attempts are made to grab a candy bar or soda.

Spices to eat

The palate often misses sugar because it has no other flavors that could replace it and many sweet tasting herbs and spices can be easily added to food and drinks to replace sugar.

Common substitutes are cinnamon, nutmeg, cardamom and vanilla. These can be added to coffee or sprinkled on oatmeal or yogurt.

Risks and considerations

Before deciding on a sugar-free diet, think twice about eliminating natural sugar. Natural sugars contained in fruits and some dairy products.

While some sugar-free diets do not allow fruit, this is not a good idea in my opinion. Fruits can contain many nutrients, fibers, antioxidants and other healthy compounds that protect the body from disease.

Fruits in a sugar-free diet can still be healthy as long as a person eats fruit in moderation.

To eliminate sugar from food, it should not be considered as a complete solution to weight loss. It should instead be part of a lifestyle change that includes regular exercise and a nutritious diet.

Anyone who wants to start a sugar-free diet should talk to a doctor or nutritionist, especially if they have health problems.

Honey

Type: A 50:50 mixture of fructose and glucose

Advantages: honey has antibacterial and antimicrobial properties, which is why it can also be used as a cough suppressant. High-quality honeys often contain healthy ingredients. On the whole, honey is more nutritious than sugar.

Disadvantage: Just as acid-forming as sugar

Our tip: If you like to eat honey, sprinkle it with a little cinnamon to counteract the acidity.

Stevia

Type: Natural replacement

Advantage: Sugar free, without calories, made from the leaves of the plant STEVIA. If you compare sweeteners with and without calories, then Stevia is at the top. It occurs naturally and is very beneficial in reasonable quantities. Natural remedy that fights inflammation.

Raw Cane Sugar

Type: sucrose

Advantages: This sugar is made from sugar cane and not refined. Also known as Turbinado sugar, it is often consumed as sugar cane juice. This is then used to sweeten nuts like almonds and cashews. It is used in many healthier recipes. This raw sugar form is slightly less processed compared to white sugar (table sugar, the most harmful kind). It still retains some of the plant's moisture and molasses, so you can technically consume fewer calories per serving.

Coconut Sugar

Type: Mainly sucrose with some nutrients

Advantages: This kind of sugar is recommended

by me. They are made from the juice of coconut palms. It is less processed. The juice is extracted and then dried, leaving it with a more natural brownish color like raw sugar. Coconut sugar contains traces of minerals such as potassium, magnesium, and inulin.

Agave Nectar

Type: More fructose than glucose (may contain up to 90% fructose)

Advantages: Tastes really good. Agave goes well with tequila (real agave is made from blue agave, like tequila) and is an integral part of margarita.

Coconut Biscuits (Small)

Ingredients

- 1 cup buckwheat groats.

- 1 cup buckwheat flour.

- 3/4 cups grated coconut.

- 2 teaspoons cinnamon.

- 1/4 teaspoon sea salt.

- 1/3 cup coconut oil, melted.

- 1/3 cup rice malt syrup.

- 1/2 teaspoon vanilla extract.

Preparation:

1. Preheat the oven to 150 ° C and line a baking sheet with parchment paper.

2. Mix the buckwheat groats, buckwheat flour, coconut, cinnamon and salt in a large bowl.

3. In a smaller bowl stir the coconut oil, rice malt syrup and vanilla extract. Pour 20ml of boiling water over the dry ingredients. Stir with a wooden spoon, until it forms a thick dough. Add more hot water if it looks a little dry.

Alternatively, if the dough is too wet, you need a little more buckwheat flour. With hands, shape the dough.

3. Shape it into flat balls and place them on the baking sheet. Bake in the oven for about 20 minutes. Let cool and place in an airtight container before serving.

Coconut Lemons Biscuits

Preparation - 10 minutes

Cooking - 20 minutes

Total - 30 minutes

Your kids will have no idea that these coconut-lemon biscuits are sugar-free because they are delicious! These nut-free cookies are filled with gelatin so that you (your children if necessary) be satisfied without making compromise with the health.

Ingredients

- 1 1/2 cup buckwheat flour.
- 1 cup of dried or shredded coconuts.
- 2 tablespoons gelatin.
- 1 teaspoon baking soda.

- 1 tablespoon ground cinnamon.

- 1/2 teaspoon sea salt.

- 125g unsalted butter (softened).

- 1 teaspoon vanilla extract.

- 1/4 cup rice malt syrup.

- 1 lemon, juice and peel.

- 1 egg.

- 1/4 cup coconut cream.

Preparation

1. Preheat the oven to 160ºC / 325ºF / gas mark 3 and lay out two baking trays with baking paper. In a large bowl, mix the buckwheat flour, gelatin powder, coconut, cinnamon, baking powder, and salt.

2. In a separate bowl, put the butter, rice malt syrup, vanilla extract, lemon juice and stir the mixture until it is creamy.

3. Add the egg and coconut cream and beat until well blended.

4. Add this mixture to the dry ingredients using a wooden spoon. The mixture should feel a bit damp, but dry enough to roll them into balls with ease.

5. Make the mixture into balls. This must be made far from the lined trays up to 4 cm. Push it down slightly. Sprinkle with a little more coconut.

6. Bake the biscuits for 20-25 minutes. The color should be golden brown. Then remove from the oven and place on a wire rack to cool. Store for up to 2 days in an airtight container.

Chocolate Cherrie Cake

Ingredients

- 2 cups almonds.

- 1/2 cup coconut.

- 1 teaspoon ground ginger.

- 100g butter (melted).

- 1 tablespoon rice malt syrup.

Filling

- 1 tablespoon gelatin.

- 1/2 cup coconut cream.

- 100g cocoa butter.

- 500g cream cheese.

- 1/3 cup rice malt syrup.

- 1/3 cup cocoa powder.

- 1 cup cherries, pitted, roughly chopped (use frozen; when out of season then replace with blueberries or raspberries).

- 100g dark chocolate, finely grated

Preparation

1. Lightly grease with butter a one springform pan. Put almonds and coconut in a blender and mix the two ingredients until they reach the consistency of almond milk. Add the ginger, rice malt syrup and melted butter. Wait for the mixture to submerge in butter and rice malt syrup.

2. Put the mixture in greased form. Put in the freezer while you are preparing the filling.

For the filling put gelatine powder and 60ml of water in a small cup or bowl. Mix until the gelatin becomes gummy. Put aside.

3. Put the coconut cream and cocoa butter in a small saucepan and heat over low heat. Heat the mixture until the cocoa butter melts. Add gelatine

and stir. Set the mixture aside and let it cool to room temperature.

4. Add the cream cheese, cocoa powder, rice malt syrup, ¾ cup of cherries and the gelatine mixture to the blender. Divide the remaining cherries into small pieces and add them to the mixture.

5. Remove the cheesecake base from the freezer and cover with the mixture. Smooth the top then leave in the fridge for at least 3 hours. Finally, sprinkle grated dark chocolate on top of cake and enjoy.

Peanut Butter Protein Pancakes

Ingredients

- 1 cup buckwheat flour.

- 1/2 cup whole wheat flour.

- 1 cup oatmeal.

- 1 teaspoon baking soda.

- 1 teaspoon sea salt.

- 1 teaspoon ground cinnamon.

- 2 tablespoons rice malt syrup.

- 1 1/4 cup whole milk.

- 1/2 teaspoon vanilla extract.

- 1/3 cup peanut butter.

- Coconut oil for frying.

Toppings:

- Mixed berries.
- Full fat or Greek yogurt or coconut yoghurt.
- Peanut butter.

Preparation

1. Mix buckwheat flour, wholegrain flour, oats, baking powder, sea salt and cinnamon in a large bowl. Add the remaining ingredients and stir until a dough forms. Put aside.

2. Heat a large pan over medium heat. Add a dollop of coconut oil, then add one cup of dough per pancake. Repeat for remaining mixture.

3. Cover the pancakes with berries, yogurt and peanut butter.

4. Vanilla Peach Kombucha

Ingredients

- 3 ½ tablespoons gelatin powder.

- 3 peaches (sliced).

- 1/4 teaspoon vanilla extract.

- 1/2 cup kombucha.

Preparation

1. Dissolve the gelatine in ⅓ cup of cold water and let it rest for few minutes then heat the peaches and vanilla in a saucepan until it becomes soft. Allow to cool slightly then blender the puree and stir in the gelatine then add the kombucha. Stir well.

2. Pour into a glass or plastic container and allow to cool. Cut into pieces and serve to enjoy delicious taste

(Tip: this dessert can be stored in an container in the refrigerator for up to 6 days).

Almond Energy Bars

Ingredients for 2 servings

- 225g gluten free oats

- 125g almond butter

- 3 scoops of chocolate protein powder

- 125ml water

- 1 teaspoon almond extract

- 1 tbsp raw cocoa powder

- 2 tbsp cocoa tips

- 3 tablespoons chia seeds

- 3 tbsp sunflower or pumpkin seeds

Preparation

1. Line a baking sheet with parchment paper. Put all dry ingredients in a blender with dough attachment and mix until smooth. Add the almond butter and the water.

2. Pour the mixture into a pan and distribute evenly. Smooth the surface. Cover and keep in the freezer for half an hour.

3. Take out and cut into bars then store the bars in the refrigerator in an airtight container.

Sugar-free Muffins

You can prepare these muffins with stevia and they will be ideal for diabetics (like all recipes). Here is the simple super recipe.

Ingredients

- 125g yoghurt
- 2 eggs
- 1 tbsp Stevia (liquid)
- 120g flour (not wheat flour)
- ½ pinch of salt
- 2 tablespoons of cocoa powder
- 1 tsp rum (flavor)
- ½ packet baking powder
- 75g chocolate sprinkles

Preparation

1. At first, mix the eggs, yogurt, and stevia then mix the flour with the salt, cocoa powder and baking powder.

2. Add the chocolate sprinkles and the rum flavor then fill muffin molds with the dough and bake at 180 ° for half an hour to enjoy delicious muffins.

Apple Pie (Autumn)

Ingredients

- 110g all-purpose wheat-free flour
- 25g gluten free oats
- 25g raisins
- 25g hazelnuts, whole
- 25g almonds, 50% chopped, 50% whole
- 1 apple, gutted and roughly chopped
- 3/4 teaspoon baking powder
- 1/2 teaspoon soda
- 1/2 tsp xanthan gum
- 1 teaspoon mixed spice (replacement: cinnamon)
- Pinch of salt
- 25g butter, margarine or low-fat spread, melted

- 100g greek yogurt or natural yoghurt

- 60ml of milk (substitute: almond, rice, soy, etc.)

- 2 tablespoons honey (substitute: agave syrup)

- 1 small egg, beaten

- 1 1/2 tsp gluten free oats (to sprinkle)

Please note that this recipe contains nuts.

Preparation

1. Preheat the oven to 200 ° C and place a cake pan with baking paper.

2. In a large bowl, mix the oats, the flour, the raisins, half the hazelnuts, the chopped almonds, apple, baking soda, baking soda, xanthine, spice mixture and salt.

3. In another bowl, mix the egg, milk, melted butter, honey and yoghurt. Pour the mixture on the dry ingredients then mix everything well.

5. Add the mixture to the mold and sprinkle with the remaining hazelnuts and almonds then add the oatmeal and bake for 40 minutes in the oven or until it turns to golden color.

Puree (mango, blueberries, avocado and peppers)

Ingredients for 2 servings

- 1/2 cup organic berries
- 1 thick slice of organic mango, peeled and diced
- 1/4 organic avocado
- 200g pepper

Preparation

1. Puree all ingredients in a blender or with a fork.

Snack with Berries and Chia Seeds

Ingredients for 2 servings

- 250g gluten free oats (normal, not flaky)
- 1 large organic apples, gutted and finely chopped
- 150g fresh blueberries
- 375ml unsweetened apple sauce
- 60g dried cranberries
- 45g unsweetened sliced coconut
- 30g of chopped walnuts
- 2 teaspoons chia seeds

Preparation

1. Preheat the oven to 180°C then line a baking pan with parchment paper. In a large bowl, put all the ingredients without the blueberries then mix well.

2. Now add the blueberries then carefully fold the mixture. Put into the baking pan and distribute evenly.

3. Bake for half an hour then remove from the oven and place on wire rack to cool.

Conclusion

All people who want to reduce their sugar intake should follow a sugar-free diet plan for whatever reason you don't want to consume sugar anymore. It may help some people to make the diet varied to easily cope with the loss of sweetness in your diet.

The elimination of sugar is probably a good idea for each person as it helps to reduce the risk of many diseases and improve the overall health of a person.